MW00575278

THE HEALTHY DIABETIC MEAL PREP COOKBOOK

AN ESSENTIAL GUIDE WITH SIMPLE AND HEALTHY RECIPES TO MANAGE DIABETES

Table of Contents

Introduction

Life with diabetes can be tough, and when you get the news you are pre-diabetic, or developed Type-2 diabetes, your whole world can be turned upside down.

One of the principal ways Type-2 diabetes can affect your life is your diet. Before you developed diabetes, chances are your diet was not a serious concern. You might have made some effort to eat healthy, or you might have enjoyed your food with no concerns.

Diabetes can be managed and treated effectively, although the process of doing so requires knowledge, discipline, patience and passion. Your health and happiness does not have to drop along with your insulin and blood glucose levels. In fact, you can make your life even better if you learn as much as you can about how your body functions as a diabetic and follow a healthy lifestyle suitable for diabetics.

Most of the successful management of diabetes relies on the right food choices, and getting enough exercise. Diabetes is a long-term condition which you will have to deal with for the rest of your life, but you can lead a full and active life when you are armed with the knowledge you need to understand and manage your condition.

Hypoglycemia is an ever-present concern for diabetics. That's when the blood sugar levels drop dangerously low, and weight loss diets and too much exercise can cause a hypoglycemic incident. In fact, just about everything about diabetes revolves around blood glucose levels, so it's important that you understand how to keep these levels stable.

Diabetes in itself is not necessarily life-threatening, but there can be complications as a result of the condition and again, most of these complications can be attributed to fluctuating blood glucose levels, which can cause a lot of stress to the system. Most of the complications associated with diabetes – including diabetic neuropathies, retinal neuropathy, heart disease, high blood pressure and high cholesterol – can be prevented or controlled by keeping blood glucose levels within the healthy range.

This book aims to provide you with simple, delicious, easy to cook meals that will be healthy for you to eat every day, as well as healthy snacks for whenever you are feeling hypo; needing sugar quickly. By sticking to five ingredients or less we make sure we always know what we are eating, and by using the Instant Pot we make sure we can cook something delicious every day.

Home Remedies To Prevent And Reverse Diabetes

There are certain things you can do at home to reduce your risk of developing diabetes or worsening it. Although you need a doctor to guide and make certain prescriptions and treatments for you, there are a lot more things you can do to manage your health as a diabetic patient. The following points below will put you on a part for better health.

- The most effective way to control and reverse diabetes is to control the food on your plate. As a diabetic, it's recommended that your home cook your meals so you can control the ingredients used for cooking.

- Consume plenty of fruits as they are rich in dietary fiber — the fruits supply energy to blood to keep your heart and organs healthy. Diabetics should limit the consumption of watermelon and pineapple because they contain have a high glycemic index of 76 GI, and 59 GI respectively, which might increase your blood sugar levels.

- Eat more non-starchy vegetables like ginger, cabbage, spinach, carrot, garlic, cucumber, onion, tomato, and radish to keep your blood sugar level at a normal range so you won't have to bother about diabetes.

- Drink plenty of plain water and avoid sugary drinks to keep your blood pressure in check.

- Avoid processed and high carb, high-calorie foods. Instead of cooking refined carbohydrate meal, choose whole grain food such as brown rice, whole wheat bread, or whole wheat pasta.

- Take a walk for about 30 minutes morning and evening thrice weekly so you can lose extra pounds weight to stay fit and keep your heart healthy.

- Get rid of fat-milk, soft drinks, and chocolate tea. Instead, drink unsweetened coffee, cocoa, or green tea without adding extra sugar. — because unsweetened coffee or tea prevents diabetes, stimulates metabolism, and helps to burn fat. So, remember to add caffeine to your shopping list.

- Reduce salt in your diet—high salt intake can increase your blood pressure. So, cook your foods by adding a pinch of salt, and a variety of other spices to make your food taste great. Do not add salt to food after cooking, or when serving at mealtime, — doing so can trigger other factors that lead to diabetes.

- Drink vegetable juice instead of sweetened fruit juice.

- Be at peace with your mind and stay stress-free. In reality, we have certain things that can bother our minds and possibly rub us of peace of mind. Sometimes, panicking affects the state of your mind and causes mental stress, which can increase your blood pressure and your total well-being. When you are in such a situation, take solace in meditation, reading spiritual books that can lift your faith, talk to your family members, and consult with your doctor.

Recipes

Breakfast

1 Steel-Cut Oatmeal Bowl with Fruit and Nuts

Preparation Time: 5 minutes
Cooking Time: 20 minutes
Servings: 4
Ingredients:
1 cup steel-cut oats
2 cups almond milk
¾ cup water
1 teaspoon ground cinnamon
¼ teaspoon salt

2 cups chopped fresh fruit, such as blueberries, strawberries, raspberries, or peaches

1/2 cup chopped walnuts

¼ cup chia seeds

Directions:

In a medium saucepan over medium-high heat, combine the oats, almond milk, water, cinnamon, and salt. Bring to a boil, reduce the heat to low, and simmer for 15 to 20 minutes, until the oats are softened and thickened.

Top each bowl with 1/2 cup of fresh fruit, 2 tablespoons of walnuts, and 1 tablespoon of chia seeds before serving.

Nutrition: Calories: 288; Total fat: 11gSaturated fat: 1gProtein: 10gCarbs: 38gSugar: 7gFiber: 10gCholesterol: 0mgSodium: 329mg

2 Whole-Grain Dutch Baby Pancake

Preparation Time: 5 minutes

Cooking Time: 25 minutes

Servings: 4

Ingredients:

2 tablespoons coconut oil

1/2 cup whole-wheat flour

¼ cup skim milk

3 large eggs

1 teaspoon vanilla extract

1/2 teaspoon baking powder

¼ teaspoon salt

¼ teaspoon ground cinnamon

Powdered sugar, for dusting

Directions:

Preheat the oven to 400F.

Put the coconut oil in a medium oven-safe skillet, and place the skillet in the oven to melt the oil while it preheats.

In a blender, combine the flour, milk, eggs, vanilla, baking powder, salt, and cinnamon. Process until smooth.

Carefully remove the skillet from the oven and tilt to spread the oil around evenly.

Pour the batter into the skillet and return it to the oven for 23 to 25 minutes, until the pancake puffs and lightly browns.

Remove, dust lightly with powdered sugar, cut into 4 wedges, and serve.

Nutrition: Calories: 195; Total fat: 11gSaturated fat: 7gProtein: 8gCarbs: 16gSugar: 1gFiber: 2gCholesterol: 140mgSodium: 209mg

3 Mushroom, Zucchini, and Onion Frittata

Preparation Time: 10 minutes

Cooking Time: 20 minutes

Servings: 4

Ingredients:

1 tablespoon extra-virgin olive oil

1/2 onion, chopped

1 medium zucchini, chopped

11/2 cups sliced mushrooms

6 large eggs, beaten

2 tablespoons skim milk

Salt

Freshly ground black pepper

1 ounce feta cheese, crumbled

Directions:

Preheat the oven to 400F.

In a medium oven-safe skillet over medium-high heat, heat the olive oil.

Add the onion and sauté for 3 to 5 minutes, until translucent.

Add the zucchini and mushrooms, and cook for 3 to 5 more minutes, until the vegetables are tender.

Meanwhile, in a small bowl, whisk the eggs, milk, salt, and pepper. Pour the mixture into the skillet, stirring to combine, and transfer the skillet to the oven. Cook for 7 to 9 minutes, until set.

Sprinkle with the feta cheese, and cook for 1 to 2 minutes more, until heated through.

Remove, cut into 4 wedges, and serve.

Nutrition: Calories: 178; Total fat: 13gSaturated fat: 4gProtein: 12gCarbs: 5gSugar: 3gFiber: 1gCholesterol: 285mgSodium: 234mg

4 Spinach and Cheese Quiche

Preparation Time: 10 minutes, plus 10 minutes to rest

Cooking Time: 50 minutes

Servings: 4 to 6

Ingredients:

Nonstick cooking spray

8 ounces Yukon Gold potatoes, shredded

1 tablespoon plus 2 teaspoons extra-virgin olive oil, divided

1 teaspoon salt, divided

Freshly ground black pepper

1 onion, finely chopped

1 (10-ounce) bag fresh spinach

4 large eggs

1/2 cup skim milk

1 ounce Gruyère cheese, shredded

Directions:

Preheat the oven to 350F. Spray a 9-inch pie dish with cooking spray. Set aside.

In a small bowl, toss the potatoes with 2 teaspoons of olive oil, 1/2 teaspoon of salt, and season with pepper. Press the potatoes into the bottom and sides of the pie dish to form a thin, even layer. Bake for 20 minutes, until golden brown. Remove from the oven and set aside to cool.

In a large skillet over medium-high heat, heat the remaining 1 tablespoon of olive oil.

Add the onion and sauté for 3 to 5 minutes, until softened.

By handfuls, add the spinach, stirring between each addition, until it just starts to wilt before adding more. Cook for about 1 minute, until it cooks down.

In a medium bowl, whisk the eggs and milk. Add the Gruyère, and season with the remaining 1/2 teaspoon of salt and some pepper. Fold the eggs into the spinach. Pour the mixture into the pie dish and bake for 25 minutes, until the eggs are set.

Let rest for 10 minutes before serving.

Nutrition: Calories: 445; Total fat: 14gSaturated fat: 4gProtein: 19gCarbs: 68gSugar: 6gFiber: 7gCholesterol: 193mgSodium: 773mg

5 Spicy Jalapeno Popper Deviled Eggs

Preparation Time: 5 minutes

Cooking Time: 5 minutes

Servings: 4

Ingredients

4 large whole eggs, hardboiled

2 tablespoons Keto-Friendly mayonnaise

¼ cup cheddar cheese, grated

2 slices bacon, cooked and crumbled

1 jalapeno, sliced

Directions:

Cut eggs in half, remove the yolk and put them in bowl

Lay egg whites on a platter

Mix in remaining ingredients and mash them with the egg yolks

Transfer yolk mix back to the egg whites

Serve and enjoy!

Nutrition: Calories: 176; Fat: 14gCarbohydrates: 0.7gProtein: 10g

6 Lovely Porridge

Preparation Time: 15 minutes

Cooking Time: Nil

Servings: 2

Ingredients

2 tablespoons coconut flour

2 tablespoons vanilla protein powder

3 tablespoons Golden Flaxseed meal

1 and 1/2 cups almond milk, unsweetened

Powdered erythritol

Directions:

Take a bowl and mix in flaxseed meal, protein powder, coconut flour and mix well

Add mix to the saucepan (placed over medium heat)

Add almond milk and stir, let the mixture thicken

Add your desired amount of sweetener and serve

Nutrition: Calories: 259; Fat: 13gCarbohydrates: 5gProtein: 16g

7 Salty Macadamia Chocolate Smoothie

Preparation Time: 5 minutes

Cooking Time: Nil

Servings: 1

Ingredients

2 tablespoons macadamia nuts, salted

1/3 cup chocolate whey protein powder, low carb

1 cup almond milk, unsweetened

Directions:

Add the listed ingredients to your blender and blend until you

have a smooth mixture

Chill and enjoy it!

Nutrition: Calories: 165; Fat: 2gCarbohydrates: 1gProtein: 12g

Meat Mains

8 Ritzy Beef Stew

Preparation time: 10 Minutes

Cooking time: 40 minutes

Servings: 6

Ingredients:

2 tablespoons all-purpose flour

1 tablespoon Italian seasoning

2 pounds (907 g) top round, cut into ¾-inch cubes

2 tablespoons olive oil

4 cups low-sodium chicken broth, divided

1½ pounds (680 g) cremini mushrooms, rinsed, stems removed, and quartered

1 large onion, coarsely chopped

3 cloves garlic, minced

3 medium carrots, peeled and cut into ½-inch pieces

1 cup frozen peas

1 tablespoon fresh thyme, minced

1 tablespoon red wine vinegar

½ teaspoon freshly ground black pepper

Directions:

Combine the flour and Italian seasoning in a large bowl. Dredge the beef cubes in the bowl to coat well.

Heat the olive oil in a pot over medium heat until shimmering.

Add the beef to the single layer in the pot and cook for 2 to 4 minutes or until golden brown on all sides. Flip the beef cubes frequently.

Remove the beef from the pot and set aside, then add ¼ cup of chicken broth to the pot.

Add the mushrooms and sauté for 4 minutes or until soft. Remove the mushrooms from the pot and set aside.

Pour ¼ cup of chicken broth in the pot. Add the onions and garlic to the pot and sauté for 4 minutes or until translucent.

Put the beef back to the pot and pour in the remaining broth. Bring to a boil.

Reduce the heat to low and cover. Simmer for 45 minutes. Stir periodically.

Add the carrots, mushroom, peas, and thyme to the pot and simmer for 45 more minutes or until the vegetables are soft.

Open the lid, drizzle with red wine vinegar and season with black pepper. Stir and serve in a large bowl.

Nutrition: calories: 250 fat: 7.0g protein: 25.0g carbs: 24.0g fiber: 3.0g sugar: 5.0g sodium: 290mg

9 Pork Trinoza Wrapped In Ham

Preparation time: 10 Minutes

Cooking time: 40 minutes

Servings: 6

Ingredients:

6 pieces of Serrano ham, thinly sliced

454g pork, halved, with butter and crushed

6g of salt

1g black pepper

227g fresh spinach leaves, divided

4 slices of mozzarella cheese, divided

18g sun-dried tomatoes, divided

10 ml of olive oil, divided

Directions:

Place 3 pieces of ham on baking paper, slightly overlapping each other. Place 1 half of the pork in the ham. Repeat with the other half.

Season the inside of the pork rolls with salt and pepper.

Place half of the spinach, cheese, and sun-dried tomatoes on top of the pork loin, leaving a 13 mm border on all sides.

Roll the fillet around the filling well and tie with a kitchen cord to keep it closed.

Repeat the process for the other pork steak and place them in the fridge.

Select Preheat in the air fryer and press Start/Pause.

Brush 5 ml of olive oil on each wrapped steak and place them in the preheated air fryer.

Select Steak. Set the timer to 9 minutes and press Start/Pause.

Allow it to cool for 10 minutes before cutting.

Nutrition: Calories: 282 Fat: 23.41 Carbohydrates: 0g Protein: 16.59 Sugar: 0g Cholesterol: 73gm

10   Mississippi Style Pot Roast

Preparation time: 10 Minutes

Cooking time: 40 minutes

Servings: 8

Ingredients:

3 lb. chuck roast

What you'll need from store cupboard:

6-8 pepperoncini

1 envelope au jus gravy mix

1 envelope ranch dressing mix

Directions:

Place roast in crock pot. Sprinkle both envelopes of mixes over top. Place the peppers around the roast.

Cover and cook on low 8 hours, or high 4 hours.

Transfer roast to a large bowl and shred using 2 forks. Add it back to the crock pot and stir. Remove the pepperoncini, chop and stir back into the roast. Serve.

Nutrition: Calories 379 Total Carbs 3g Protein 56g Fat 14g Sugar 1g Fiber 0g

11   Spicy Grilled Turkey Breast

Preparation time: 10 Minutes

Cooking time: 40 minutes

Servings: 14

Ingredients:

5 lb. turkey breast, bone in

What you'll need from store cupboard:

1 cup low sodium chicken broth

¼ cup vinegar

¼ cup jalapeno pepper jelly

2 tbsp. Splenda brown sugar

2 tbsp. olive oil

1 tbsp. salt

2 tsp cinnamon

1 tsp cayenne pepper

½ tsp ground mustard

Nonstick cooking spray

Directions:

Heat grill to medium heat. Spray rack with cooking spray. Place a drip pan on the grill for indirect heat.

In a small bowl, combine Splenda brown sugar with seasonings.

Carefully loosen the skin on the turkey from both sides with your fingers. Spread half the spice mix on the turkey. Secure the skin to the underneath with toothpicks and spread remaining spice mix on the outside.

Place the turkey over the drip pan and grill 30 minutes.

In a small saucepan, over medium heat, combine broth, vinegar, jelly, and oil. Cook and stir 2 minutes until jelly is completely melted. Reserve ½ cup of the mixture.

Baste turkey with some of the jelly mixture. Cook 1-1 ½ hours, basting every 15 minutes, until done, when thermometer reaches 170 degrees.

Cover and let rest 10 minutes. Discard the skin. Brush with reserved jelly mixture and slice and serve.

Nutrition: Calories 314 Total Carbs 5g Protein 35g Fat 14g Sugar 5g Fiber 0g

12   Stuffed Cabbage And Pork Loin Rolls

Preparation time: 10 Minutes

Cooking time: 40 minutes

Servings: 4

Ingredients:

500g of white cabbage

1 onion

8 pork tenderloin steaks

2 carrots

4 tbsp. soy sauce

50g of olive oil

Salt

8 sheets of rice

Directions:

Put the chopped cabbage in the Thermo mix glass together with the onion and the chopped carrot.

Select 5 seconds, speed 5. Add the extra virgin olive oil. Select 5 minutes, varoma temperature, left turn, spoon speed.

Cut the tenderloin steaks into thin strips. Add the meat to the Thermomix glass. Select 5 minutes, varoma temperature, left turn, spoon speed. Without beaker

Add the soy sauce. Select 5 minutes, varoma temperature, left turn, spoon speed. Rectify salt. Let it cold down.

Hydrate the rice slices. Extend and distribute the filling between them.

Make the rolls, folding so that the edges are completely closed. Place the rolls in the air fryer and paint with the oil. Select 10 minutes, 1800C.

Nutrition: Calories: 120 Fat: 3.41g Carbohydrates: 0g Protein: 20.99g Sugar: 0gCholesterol: 65mg

13   Cherry Apple Pork

Preparation time: 10 minutes

Cooking time: 30 minutes

Servings: 2

Ingredients:

Apple (1 small, diced)

Cherries (.3 c pitted)

Onion (3 T diced)

Celery (3 T diced)

Apple juice (.25 c)

Black pepper

Pork loin (.75 lb.)

Water (.25 c)

Directions:

Add all of the ingredients to the Instant Pot cooker and mix thoroughly.

Seal the lid of the cooker, choose the poultry setting and set the time for 5 minutes.

Once the timer goes off, select the quick pressure release option and remove the lid as soon as the pressure has normalized.

Serve warm.

Nutrition: Protein: 12 grams Carbs: 22.9 grams Fiber: 19 grams Sugar: 11.2 grams Fats: 28 grams Calories: 453

Seafood

14   Tilapia with Lemon Garlic Sauce

Preparation Time: 15 minutes

Cooking Time: 30 minutes

Servings: 4

Ingredients:

Pepper

1 teaspoon dried parsley flakes

1 clove garlic (finely chopped)

1 tablespoon butter (melted)

3 tablespoons. fresh lemon juice

4 tilapia fillets

Directions:

First, spray baking dish with non-stick cooking spray then preheat oven at 375 degrees Fahrenheit (190oC).

In cool water, rinse tilapia fillets and using paper towels pat dry the fillets.

Place tilapia fillets in the baking dish then pour butter and lemon juice and top off with pepper, parsley and garlic.

Bake tilapia in the preheated oven for 30 minutes and wait until fish is white.

Enjoy!

Nutrition:

Calories:168;

Carbs: 4g

Protein: 24g

Fats: 5g

Phosphorus: 207mg

Potassium: 431mg

Sodium: 85mg

15   Lemon Butter Salmon

Preparation Time: 15 minutes

Cooking Time: 15 minutes

Servings: 6

Ingredients:

1 tablespoon butter

2 tablespoons olive oil

1 tablespoon Dijon mustard

1 tablespoons lemon juice

2 cloves garlic, crushed

1 teaspoon dried dill

1 teaspoon dried basil leaves

1 tablespoon capers

24-ounce salmon filet

Directions:

Put all of the ingredients except the salmon in a saucepan over medium heat.

Bring to a boil and then simmer for 5 minutes.

Preheat your grill.

Create a packet using foil.

Place the sauce and salmon inside.

Seal the packet.

Grill for 12 minutes.

Nutrition:

Calories 292

Protein 22 g

Carbohydrates 2 g

Fat 22 g

Cholesterol 68 mg

Sodium 190 mg

Potassium 439 mg

Phosphorus 280 mg

Calcium 21 mg

16   Crab Cake

Preparation Time: 15 minutes

Cooking Time: 9 minutes

Servings: 6

Ingredients:

1/4 cup onion, chopped

1/4 cup bell pepper, chopped

1 egg, beaten

6 low-sodium crackers, crushed

1/4 cup low-fat mayonnaise

1-pound crab meat

1 tablespoon dry mustard

Pepper to taste

2 tablespoons lemon juice

1 tablespoon fresh parsley

1 tablespoon garlic powder

3 tablespoons olive oil

Directions:

Mix all the ingredients except the oil.

Form 6 patties from the mixture.

Pour the oil into a pan in a medium heat.

Cook the crab cakes for 5 minutes.

Flip and cook for another 4 minutes.

Nutrition:

Calories 189

Protein 13 g

Carbohydrates 5 g

Fat 14 g

Cholesterol 111 mg

Sodium 342 mg

Potassium 317 mg

Phosphorus 185 mg

Calcium 52 mg

Fiber 0.5 g

17   Baked Fish in Cream Sauce

Preparation Time: 10 minutes

Cooking Time: 40 minutes

Servings: 4

Ingredients:

1-pound haddock

1/2 cup all-purpose flour

2 tablespoons butter (unsalted)

1/4 teaspoon pepper

2 cups fat-free nondairy creamer

1/4 cup water

Directions:

Preheat your oven to 350 degrees F.

Spray baking pan with oil.

Sprinkle with a little flour.

Arrange fish on the pan

Season with pepper.

Sprinkle remaining flour on the fish.

Spread creamer on both sides of the fish.

Bake for 40 minutes or until golden.

Spread cream sauce on top of the fish before serving.

Nutrition:

Calories 383

Protein 24 g

Carbohydrates 46 g

Fat 11 g

Cholesterol 79 mg

Sodium 253 mg

Potassium 400 mg

Phosphorus 266 mg

Calcium 46 mg

Fiber 0.4 g

18   Shrimp & Broccoli

Preparation Time: 10 minutes

Cooking Time: 5 minutes

Servings: 4

Ingredients:

1 tablespoon olive oil

1 clove garlic, minced

1-pound shrimp

1/4 cup red bell pepper

1 cup broccoli florets, steamed

10-ounce cream cheese

1/2 teaspoon garlic powder

1/4 cup lemon juice

3/4 teaspoon ground peppercorns

1/4 cup half and half creamer

Directions:

Pour the oil and cook garlic for 30 seconds.

Add shrimp and cook for 2 minutes.

Add the rest of the ingredients.

Mix well.

Cook for 2 minutes.

Nutrition:

Calories 469

Protein 28 g

Carbohydrates 28 g

Fat 28 g

Cholesterol 213 mg

Sodium 374 mg

Potassium 469 mg

Phosphorus 335 mg

Calcium 157 mg

Fiber 2.6 g

19   Fish with Mushrooms

Preparation Time: 5 minutes

Cooking Time: 16 minutes

Servings: 4

Ingredients:

1-pound cod fillet

2 tablespoons butter

¼ cup white onion, chopped

1 cup fresh mushrooms

1 teaspoon dried thyme

Directions:

Put the fish in a baking pan.

Preheat your oven to 450 degrees F.

Melt the butter and cook onion and mushroom for 1 minute.

Spread mushroom mixture on top of the fish.

Season with thyme.

Bake in the oven for 15 minutes.

Nutrition:

Calories 156

Protein 21 g

Carbohydrates 3 g

Fat 7 g

Cholesterol 49 mg

Sodium 110 mg

Potassium 561 mg

Phosphorus 225 mg

Calcium 30 mg

Fiber 0.5 g

Poultry

20   Lemon Chicken With Basil

Preparation time: 10 minutes

Cooking time: 30 minutes

Servings: 4

Ingredients:

1kg chopped chicken

1 or 2 lemons

Basil, salt, and ground pepper

Extra virgin olive oil

Directions:

Put the chicken in a bowl with a jet of extra virgin olive oil.

Put salt, pepper, and basil.

Bind well and let stand for at least 30 minutes stirring occasionally.

Put the pieces of chicken in the air fryer basket and take the air fryer

Select 30 minutes.

Occasionally remove.

Take out and put another batch.

Do the same operation.

Nutrition: Calories: 126 Fat: 6g Carbohydrates 0g Protein: 18g Sugar: 0g

21   Chicken, Oats & Chickpeas Meatloaf

Preparation time: 10 minutes

Cooking time: 30 minutes

Servings: 4

Ingredients:

½ cup cooked chickpeas

2 egg whites

2½ teaspoons poultry seasoning

Ground black pepper, as required

10 ounce lean ground chicken

1 cup red bell pepper, seeded and minced

1 cup celery stalk, minced

1/3 cup steel-cut oats

1 cup tomato puree, divided

2 tablespoons dried onion flakes, crushed

1 tablespoon prepared mustard

Directions:

Preheat the oven to 350 degrees F. Grease a 9x5-inch loaf pan.

In a food processor, add chickpeas, egg whites, poultry seasoning and black pepper and pulse until smooth.

Transfer the mixture into a large bowl.

Add the chicken, veggies oats, ½ cup of tomato puree and onion flakes and mix until well combined.

Transfer the mixture into prepared loaf pan evenly.

With your hands, press, down the mixture slightly.

In another bowl mix together mustard and remaining tomato puree.

Place the mustard mixture over loaf pan evenly.

Bake for about 1-1¼ hours or until desired doneness.

Remove from the oven and set aside for about 5 minutes before slicing.g.

Cut into desired sized slices and serve.

Meal Prep Tip: In a resealable plastic bag, place the cooled meatloaf slices and seal the bag. Refrigerate for about 2-4 days. Reheat in the microwave on High for about 1 minute before serving.

Nutrition: Calories 229 Total Fat 5.6 g Saturated Fat 1.4 g Cholesterol 50 mg Total Carbs 23.7 g Sugar 5.2 g Fiber 4.7 g Sodium 227 mg Potassium 509 mg Protein 21.4 g

22   Turkey Stuffed Poblano Peppers

Preparation time: 10 Minutes

Cooking time: 40 minutes

Servings: 2

Ingredients:

2 Poblano peppers, halved lengthwise, cores and seeds removed

1 lb. ground turkey

½ cup low-fat cheddar cheese, grated

1 green onion, diced

1 tbsp. cilantro, chopped

What you'll need from store cupboard:

8 oz. can tomato sauce

1 tbsp. olive oil

1 tsp oregano

1 tsp paprika

1 tsp ground cumin

½ tsp onion powder

½ tsp garlic paste or minced garlic

Salt and pepper

Directions:

Heat oven to 350 degrees.

Use tongs to roast the skin of the peppers over an open flame until charred and blistered all over. Or place on a cookie sheet under the broiler until skin is charred.

Place peppers in a plastic bag to steam for 15 minutes.

In a small bowl, stir together tomato sauce, oregano, paprika, and cumin

Heat oil in a large skillet over medium heat. Add turkey, onion powder, and garlic paste. Cook, stirring frequently, until meat has browned. Stir in 2 tablespoons of the sauce and season with salt and pepper.

Pour remaining sauce in the bottom of a baking dish.

With a butter knife, scrape the charred skin off the peppers, and place on sauce in dish.

Divide turkey mixture evenly over the peppers, sprinkle with cheese. Cover and bake 20 minutes.

Remove the foil, and bake until cheese starts to brown, about 5-7 minutes. Serve garnished with chopped green onion and cilantro.

Nutrition: Calories 665 Total Carbs 12g Net Carbs 9g Protein 71g Fat 36g Sugar 8g Fiber 3g

23   Hearty Beef Chili

Preparation time: 10 Minutes

Cooking time: 40 minutes

Servings: 4

Ingredients:

1 lb. lean ground beef

1 large bell pepper, diced

1 cup onion, diced

What you'll need from store cupboard:

4 oz. can green chilies, diced

1 cup tomato sauce

1 cup low sodium beef broth

1 tbsp. tomato paste

2 cloves garlic, diced fine

2 tsp chili powder

1 tsp salt

1 tsp Worcestershire

1 tsp cumin

½ tsp celery salt

¼ tsp pepper

Directions:

Heat a large pan over med-high heat. Add beef, onions, bell pepper and garlic and cook, stirring occasionally, until beef is no longer pink. Drain fat.

Add remaining Ingredients and bring to a simmer. Reduce heat to med-low and simmer 30 minutes to an hour. Taste and adjust seasonings if needed. Serve.

Nutrition: Calories 355 Total Carbs 30g Net Carbs 20g Protein 40g Fat 9g Sugar 18g Fiber 10g

24   Turkey Sloppy Joes

Preparation time: 10 Minutes

Cooking time: 40 minutes

Servings: 8

Ingredients:

1 lb. lean ground turkey

1 onion, diced

½ cup celery, diced

¼ cup green bell pepper, diced

What you'll need from store cupboard:

8 Flourless Burger Buns

1 can no salt added condensed tomato soup

½ cup ketchup

2 tbsp. yellow mustard

1 tbsp. Splenda brown sugar

¼ tsp pepper

Directions:

In a large saucepan, over medium heat, cook turkey, onion, celery, and green pepper until turkey is no longer pink. Transfer to crock pot.

Add remaining Ingredients and stir to combine. Cover, and cook on low heat 4 hours. Stir well and serve on buns.

Nutrition: Calories 197 Total Carbs 12g Net Carbs 11g Protein 17g Fat 8g Sugar 8g Fiber 1g

25   Chestnut Stuffed Pork Roast

Preparation time: 10 Minutes

Cooking time: 40 minutes

Servings: 15

Ingredients:

5 lb. pork loin roast, boneless, double tied

½ lb. ground pork

½ cup celery, diced fine

½ cup onion, diced fine

2 tbsp. fresh parsley, diced, divided

1 tbsp. margarine

What you'll need from store cupboard:

15 oz. can chestnuts, drained

2 cup low sodium chicken broth

3 tbsp. flour

2 tbsp. brandy, divided

½ tsp salt

½ tsp pepper

1/8 tsp allspice

Salt & black pepper, to taste

Directions:

Heat oven to 350 degrees.

Untie roast, open and pound lightly to even thickness.

Melt margarine in a skillet over med-high heat. Add celery and onion and cook until soft.

In a large bowl, combine ground pork, 1 tablespoon parsley, 1 tablespoon brandy and seasonings. Mix in celery and onion. Spread over roast.

Lay a row of chestnuts down the center. Roll meat around filling and tie securely with butcher string. Roast in oven 1 ½ hours or until meat thermometer reaches 145 degrees. Remove and let rest 10 minutes.

Measure out 2 tablespoons of drippings, discard the rest, into a saucepan. Place over medium heat and whisk in flour until smooth. Add broth and cook, stirring, until mixture thickens. Chop remaining chestnuts and add to gravy along with remaining brandy and parsley. Season with salt and pepper if desired. Slice the roast and serve topped with gravy.

Nutrition: Calories 416 Total Carbs 15g Protein 48g Fat 16g Sugar 0g Fiber 0g

Vegetarian and Vegan

26   Kale With Miso & Ginger

Preparation time: 10 minutes

Cooking time: 30 minutes

Servings: 6

Ingredients:

8 oz. fresh kale, sliced into strips

1 clove garlic, minced

1 tablespoon lime juice

½ teaspoon lime zest

2 tablespoons oil

2 tablespoons rice vinegar

1 teaspoon fresh ginger, grated

2 teaspoons miso

2 tablespoons dry roasted cashews, chopped

Directions:

Steam kale on a steamer basket in a pot with water.

Transfer kale to a bowl.

Mix the rest of the ingredients except cashews in another bowl.

Toss kale in the mixture.

Top with chopped cashews before serving.

Nutrition: Calories 86 Total Fat 5 g Saturated Fat 0 g Cholesterol 0 mg Sodium 104 mg Total Carbohydrate 9 g Dietary Fiber 2 g Total Sugars 2 g Protein 3 g Potassium 352 mg

27   Beans, Walnuts & Veggie Burgers

Preparation time: 10 minutes

Cooking time: 30 minutes

Servings: 8

Ingredients:

½ cup walnuts

1 carrot, peeled and chopped

1 celery stalk, chopped

4 scallions, chopped

5 garlic cloves, chopped

2¼ cups cooked black beans

2½ cups sweet potato, peeled and grated

½ teaspoon red pepper flakes, crushed

¼ teaspoon cayenne pepper

Salt and ground black pepper, as required

Directions:

Preheat the oven to 400 degrees F. Line a baking sheet with parchment paper.

In a food processor, add walnuts and pulse until finely ground.

Add the carrot, celery, scallion and garlic and pulse until chopped finely.

Transfer the vegetable mixture into a large bowl.

In the same food processor, add beans and pulse until chopped.

Add 1½ cups of sweet potato and pulse until a chunky mixture forms.

Transfer the bean mixture into the bowl with vegetable mixture.

Stir in the remaining sweet potato and spices and mix until well combined.

Make 8 patties from mixture.

Arrange the patties onto prepared baking sheet in a single layer.

Bake for about 25 minutes.

Serve hot.

Nutrition: Calories 177 Total Fat 5 g Saturated Fat 0.3 g Cholesterol 0 mg Total Carbs 27.6 g Sugar 5.3 g Fiber 7.6 g Sodium 205 mg Potassium 398 mg Protein 8 g

28 Artichoke Quiche

Preparation time: 10 minutes

Cooking time: 30 minutes

Servings: 6

Ingredients:

2 cups long-grain rice, cooked

¾ cup egg substitute

¼ cup green onions, sliced

¼ teaspoon white pepper, ground

1 can artichoke hearts

What you will need from the store cupboard:

¾ cup low-fat cheddar cheese

1 garlic clove, crushed

¾ cup fat-free milk

½ teaspoon salt

1 tablespoon Dijon mustard

Cooking spray

Directions:

Bring together the egg substitute, ¼ cup cheese, garlic, salt, and rice.

Apply cooking spray to a pie plate. Bake for 5 minutes.

Keep the artichoke quarters at the bottom of your rice crust.

Now sprinkle the remaining cheese.

Combine the remaining milk, egg substitute, and the other ingredients.

Pour the cheese over.

Bake until it sets.

Cut into wedges and garnish with the onion strips.

Nutrition: Calories 169, Carbohydrates 23g, Fiber 1g, Cholesterol 11mg, Fat 4g, Protein 10g, Sodium 490mg

Preparation time: 10 minutes

Cooking time: 30 minutes

Servings: 4

Ingredients:

2 tablespoons olive oil

1 cup quinoa, rinsed

1 green bell pepper, seeded and chopped

1 medium onion, chopped finely

3 garlic cloves, minced

2½ cups filtered water

2 cups tomatoes, crushed finely

1 teaspoon red chili powder

¼ teaspoon ground cumin

¼ teaspoon garlic powder

Ground black pepper, as required

Directions:

In a large pan, heat the oil over medium-high heat and cook the quinoa, onion, bell pepper and garlic for about 5 minutes, stirring frequently.

Stir in the remaining ingredients and bring to a boil.

Now, reduce the heat to medium-low.

Cover the pan tightly and simmer for about 3o minutes, stirring occasionally.

Serve hot.

Meal Prep Tip: Transfer the quinoa mixture into a large bowl and set aside to cool. Divide the chili into 4 containers evenly. Cover the containers and refrigerate for 1-2 days. Reheat in the microwave before serving.

Nutrition: Calories 260 Total Fat 10 g Saturated Fat 1.4 g Cholesterol 0 mg Total Carbs 36.9 g Sugar 5.2 g Fiber 5.4 g Sodium 16 mg Potassium 575 mg Protein 7.7 g

30   Black Bean With Poblano Tortilla Wraps

Preparation time: 10 minutes

Cooking time: 30 minutes

Servings: 4

Ingredients:

½ teaspoon cumin, ground

1/3 cup poblano chili, chopped

1 cup avocado, diced and peeled

¼ cup red onion, chopped

1 can rinse and drained black beans

What you will need from the store cupboard:

½ cup low-fat sour cream

3 tablespoons lime juice

4 flour tortillas

¼ teaspoon salt

Directions:

Combine the cumin and sour cream in a bowl. Use a whisk to stir.

Bring together the beans and other ingredients.

Spoon out the mixture at the center of the tortillas.

Roll them up. Cut through the middle.

Use wooden picks to secure.

Serve with your sour cream mixture.

Nutrition: Calories 298, Carbohydrates 40g, Fiber 5g, Cholesterol 16mg, Fat 13g, Protein 9g, Sodium 606mg

31   Mixed Greens Salad

Preparation time: 10 minutes

Cooking time: 30 minutes

Servings: 6

Ingredients:

6 cups mixed salad greens

1 cup cucumber, chopped

½ cup carrot, shredded

¼ cup bell pepper, sliced into strips

¼ cup cherry tomatoes, sliced in half

6 tablespoons white onion, chopped

6 tablespoons balsamic vinaigrette dressing

Directions:

Toss all the ingredients in a large salad bowl.

Drizzle dressing on top or serve on the side.

Nutrition: Calories 23 Total Fat 1 g Saturated Fat 0 g Cholesterol 0 mg Sodium 138 mg Total Carbohydrate 4 g Dietary Fiber 1 g Total Sugars 1 g Protein 1 g Potassium 142 mg

32   Tofu Curry

Preparation time: 10 minutes

Cooking time: 30 minutes

Servings: 2

Ingredients:

2 cups cubed extra firm tofu

2 cups mixed stir fry vegetables

0.5 cup soy yogurt

3tbsp curry paste

1tbsp oil or ghee

Directions:

Set the Instant Pot to saute and add the oil and curry paste.

When the onion is soft, add the remaining ingredients except the yogurt and seal.

Cook on Stew for 20 minutes.

Release the pressure naturally and serve with a scoop of soy yogurt.

Nutrition: Calories: 300 Carbs: 9 Sugar: 4 Fat: 14 Protein: 42 GL: 7

33   Baked Beans

Preparation time: 10 minutes

Cooking time: 30 minutes

Servings: 6

Ingredients:

2 cups navy beans, overnight soaked in cold water

2/3 cups green bell pepper, diced

1 can tomatoes, diced

1 onion, sliced

What you will need from the store cupboard:

3 tablespoons molasses

¼ cup of orange juice

¼ cup maple syrup

1 tablespoon Worcestershire sauce

1/4 teaspoon mustard powder

2 tablespoons stevia sugar

2 tablespoons salt

Directions:

Preheat your oven to 350 °F

Simmer the beans. Drain and keep the liquid.

Place beans in a casserole dish with the onion.

Bring together the dry mustard, pepper, salt, molasses, Worcestershire sauce, tomatoes, sugar substitute and orange juice in your saucepan.

Boil the mix. Pour over your beans.

Pour the reserved bean water, covering the beans.

Use aluminum foil to cover the dish.

Now bake in the oven. The beans must get tender.

Remove the foil and add some liquid if needed.

Nutrition: Calories 482, Carbohydrates 65g, Cholesterol 25mg, Fiber 12g, Fat 16g, Protein 21g, Sugar 2.2g, Sodium 512mg

34   Spicy Black Beans

Preparation time: 10 minutes

Cooking time: 30 minutes

Servings: 6

Ingredients:

4 cups filtered water

1½ cups dried black beans, soaked for 8 hours and drained

½ teaspoon ground turmeric

3 tablespoons olive oil

1 small onion, chopped finely

1 green chili, chopped

1 (1-inch) piece fresh ginger, minced

2 garlic cloves, minced

1-1½ tablespoons ground coriander

1 teaspoon ground cumin

½ teaspoon cayenne pepper

Sea salt, as required

2 medium tomatoes, chopped finely

½ cup fresh cilantro, chopped

Directions:

In a large pan, add water, black beans and turmeric and bring to a boil on high heat.

Now, reduce the heat to low and simmer, covered for about 1 hour or till desired doneness of beans.

Meanwhile, in a skillet, heat the oil over medium heat and sauté the onion for about 4-5 minutes.

Add the green chili, ginger, garlic, spices and salt and sauté for about 1-2 minutes.

Stir in the tomatoes and cook for about 10 minutes, stirring occasionally.

Transfer the tomato mixture into the pan with black beans and stir to combine.

Increase the heat to medium-low and simmer for about 15-20 minutes.

Stir in the cilantro and simmer for about 5 minutes.

Serve hot.

Meal Prep Tip: Transfer the beans mixture into a large bowl and set aside to cool. Divide the mixture into 6 containers evenly. Cover the containers and refrigerate for 1-2 days. Reheat in the microwave before serving.

Nutrition: Calories 160 Total Fat 8 g Saturated Fat 1 g Cholesterol 0 mg Total Carbs 17.9 g Sugar 2.4 g Fiber 6.2 g Sodium 50 mg Potassium 343 mg Protein 6 g

35   Cauliflower Mushroom Risotto

Preparation time: 10 minutes

Cooking time: 30 minutes

Servings: 2

Ingredients:

1 medium head cauliflower, grated

8-ounce Porcini mushrooms, sliced

1 yellow onion, diced fine

2 cup low sodium vegetable broth

2 teaspoon garlic, diced fine

2 teaspoon white wine vinegar

Salt & pepper, to taste

Olive oil cooking spray

Directions:

Heat oven to 350 degrees. Line a baking sheet with foil. Place the mushrooms on the prepared pan and spray with cooking spray. Sprinkle with salt and toss to coat. Bake 10-12 minutes, or until golden brown and the mushrooms start to crisp.

Spray a large skillet with cooking spray and place over med-high heat. Add onion and cook, stirring frequently, until translucent, about 3-4 minutes. Add garlic and cook 2 minutes, until golden.

Add the cauliflower and cook 1 minute, stirring.

Place the broth in a saucepan and bring to a simmer. Add to the skillet, ¼ cup at a time, mixing well after each addition. Stir in vinegar. Reduce heat to low and let simmer, 4-5 minutes, or until most of the liquid has evaporated.

Spoon cauliflower mixture onto plates, or in bowls, and top with mushrooms. Serve.

Nutrition: Calories 134 Total Carbohydrates 22g Protein 10g Fat 0g Sugar 5g Fiber 2g

---

Salads, Sauces, Dressings & Dips

36   Garden Wraps

Preparation Time: 20 minutes

Cooking Time: 10 minutes

Servings: 8

Ingredients:

1 cucumber, chopped

1 sweet corn

1 cabbage, shredded

1 tablespoon lettuce, minced

1 tomato, chopped

What you will need from the store cupboard:

3 tablespoons of rice vinegar

2 teaspoons peanut butter

1/3 cup onion paste

1/3 cup chili sauce

2 teaspoons of low-sodium soy sauce

Directions:

Cut corn from the cob. Keep in a bowl.

Add the tomato, cabbage, cucumber, and onion paste.

Now whisk the vinegar, peanut butter, and chili sauce together.

Pour this over the vegetable mix. Toss for coating.

Let this stand for 10 minutes.

Take your slotted spoon and place 1/2 cup salad in every lettuce leaf.

Fold the lettuce over your filling.

Nutrition: Calories 64, Carbs 13g, Fiber 2g, Sugar 1g, Cholesterol 0mg, Total Fat 1g, Protein 2g

37   Party Shrimp

Preparation Time: 15 minutes

Cooking Time: 10 minutes

Servings: 30

Ingredients:

16 oz. uncooked shrimp, peeled and deveined

1-1/2 teaspoons of juice from a lemon

1/2 teaspoon basil, chopped

1 teaspoon coriander, chopped

1/2 cup tomato

What you will need from the store cupboard:

1 tablespoon of olive oil

1/2 teaspoon Italian seasoning

1/2 teaspoon paprika

1 sliced garlic clove

¼ teaspoon pepper

Directions:

Bring together everything except the shrimp in a dish or bowl.

Add the shrimp. Coat well by tossing. Set aside.

Drain the shrimp. Discard the marinade.

Keep them on a baking sheet. It should not be greased.

Broil each side for 4 minutes. The shrimp should become pink.

Nutrition: Calories 14, Carbs 0g, Fiber 0g, Sugar 0g,

Cholesterol 18mg, Total Fat 0g, Protein 2g

38   Creamy Crab Slaw

Preparation time: 10 minutes, chill time: 1 hour

Servings: 4

Ingredients:

½ lb. cabbage, shredded

½ lb. red cabbage, shredded

2 hard-boiled eggs, chopped

Juice of 1/2 lemon

What you'll need from store cupboard:

2 6 oz. cans crabmeat, drained

½ cup lite mayonnaise

1 tsp celery seeds

Salt & pepper, to taste

Directions:

In a large bowl, combine both kinds of cabbage.

In a small bowl, combine mayonnaise, lemon juice, and celery seeds. Add to cabbage and toss to coat.

Add crab and eggs and toss to mix, season with salt and pepper. Cover and refrigerate 1 hour before serving.

Nutrition:

Calories 380 Total Carbs 25g Net Carbs 17g Protein 18g Fat 24g Sugar 13g Fiber 8g

39   Festive Holiday Salad

Preparation time: 10 minutes, chill time: 1 hour

Servings: 8

Ingredients:

1 head broccoli, separated into florets

1 head cauliflower, separated into florets

1 red onion, sliced thin

2 cup cherry tomatoes, halved

½ cup fat free sour cream

What you'll need from store cupboard:

1 cup lite mayonnaise

1 tbsp. Splenda

Directions:

In a large bowl combine vegetables.

In a small bowl, whisk together mayonnaise, sour cream and Splenda. Pour over vegetables and toss to mix.

Cover and refrigerate at least 1 hour before serving.

Nutrition:

Calories 152 Total Carbs 12g Net Carbs 10g Protein 2g Fat 10g Sugar 5g Fiber 2g

40   Grilled Vegetable & Noodle Salad

Preparation time: 15 minutes

Cooking time: 10 minutes

Servings: 4

Ingredients:

2 ears corn-on-the-cob, husked

1 red onion, cut in ½-inch thick slices

1 tomato, diced fine

1/3 cup fresh basil, diced

1/3 cup feta cheese, crumbled

What you'll need from store cupboard:

1 recipe Homemade Noodles, cook & drain

4 tbsp. Herb Vinaigrette

Nonstick cooking spray

Directions:

Heat grill to medium heat. Spray rack with cooking spray. Place corn and onions on the grill and cook, turning when needed, until lightly charred and tender, about 10 minutes. Cut corn off the cob and place in a medium bowl. Chop the onion and add to the corn.

Stir in noodles, tomatoes, basil, and vinaigrette, toss to mix. Sprinkle cheese over top and serve.

Nutrition:

Calories 330 Total Carbs 19g Net Carbs 16g Protein 10g Fat 9g Sugar 5g Fiber 3g

41   Harvest Salad

Preparation time: 15 minutes

Cooking time: 25 minutes

Servings: 6

Ingredients:

10 oz. kale, deboned and chopped

1 ½ cup blackberries

½ butternut squash, cubed

¼ cup goat cheese, crumbled

What you'll need from store cupboard:

Maple Mustard Salad Dressing

1 cup raw pecans

1/3 cup raw pumpkin seeds

¼ cup dried cranberries

3 1/2 tbsp. olive oil

1 ½ tbsp. sugar free maple syrup

3/8 tsp salt, divided

Pepper, to taste

Nonstick cooking spray

Directions:

Heat oven to 400 degrees. Spray a baking sheet with cooking spray.

Spread squash on the prepared pan, add 1 ½ tablespoons oil, 1/8 teaspoon salt, and pepper to squash and stir to coat the squash evenly. Bake 20-25 minutes.

Place kale in a large bowl. Add 2 tablespoons oil and ½ teaspoon salt and massage it into the kale with your hands for 3-4 minutes.

Spray a clean baking sheet with cooking spray. In a medium bowl, stir together pecans, pumpkin seeds, and maple syrup until nuts are coated. Pour onto prepared pan and bake 8-10 minutes, these can be baked at the same time as the squash.

To assemble the salad: place all of the Ingredients in a large bowl. Pour dressing over and toss to coat. Serve.

Nutrition:

Calories 436 Total Carbs 24g Net Carbs 17g Protein 9g Fat 37g Sugar 5g Fiber 7g

---

Dessert and Snacks

42   Chocolate Chip Blondies

Preparation time: 5 minutes

Cooking time: 20 minutes

Servings: 12

Ingredients:

1 egg

What you'll need from store cupboard:

½ cup semisweet chocolate chips

1/3 cup flour

1/3 cup whole wheat flour

¼ cup Splenda brown sugar

¼ cup sunflower oil

2 tbsp. honey

1 tsp vanilla

½ tsp baking powder

¼ tsp salt

Nonstick cooking spray

Directions:

Heat oven to 350 degrees. Spray an 8-inch square baking dish with cooking spray.

In a small bowl, combine dry Ingredients.

In a large bowl, whisk together egg, oil, honey, and vanilla. Stir in dry Ingredients just until combined. Stir in chocolate chips.

Spread batter in prepared dish. Bake 20-22 minutes or until they pass the toothpick test. Cool on a wire rack then cut into bars.

Nutrition:

Calories 136 Total Carbs 18g Net Carbs 16g Protein 2g Fat 6g Sugar 9g Fiber 2g

43   Cinnamon Apple Chips

Preparation time: 5 minutes

Cooking time: 10 minutes

Servings: 2

Ingredients:

1 medium apple, sliced thin

What you'll need from store cupboard:

¼ tsp cinnamon

¼ tsp nutmeg

Nonstick cooking spray

Directions:

Heat oven to 375. Spray a baking sheet with cooking spray.

Place apples in a mixing bowl and add spices. Toss to coat.
Arrange apples, in a single layer, on prepared pan. Bake 4
minutes, turn apples over and bake 4 minutes more.

Serve immediately or store in airtight container.

Nutrition:

Calories 58 Total Carbs 15g Protein 0g Fat 0g Sugar 11g Fiber
3g

44   Cinnamon Apple Popcorn

Preparation time: 30 minutes

Cooking time: 50 minutes

Servings: 11

Ingredients:

4 tbsp. margarine, melted

What you'll need from store cupboard

10 cup plain popcorn

2 cup dried apple rings, unsweetened and chopped

½ cup walnuts, chopped

2 tbsp. Splenda brown sugar

1 tsp cinnamon

½ tsp vanilla

Directions:

Heat oven to 250 degrees.

Place chopped apples in a 9x13-inch baking dish and bake 20
minutes. Remove from oven and stir in popcorn and nuts.

In a small bowl, whisk together margarine, vanilla, Splenda, and cinnamon. Drizzle evenly over popcorn and toss to coat. Bake 30 minutes, stirring quickly every 10 minutes. If apples start to turn a dark brown, remove immediately.

Pout onto waxed paper to cool at least 30 minutes. Store in an airtight container. Serving size is 1 cup.

Nutrition:

Calories 133 Total Carbs 14g Net Carbs 11g Protein 3g Fat 8g Sugar 7g Fiber 3g

45   Crab & Spinach Dip

Preparation time: 10 minutes

Cooking time: 2 hours

Servings: 10

Ingredients:

1 pkg. frozen chopped spinach, thawed and squeezed nearly dry

8 oz. reduced-fat cream cheese

What you'll need from store cupboard:

6 ½ oz. can crabmeat, drained and shredded

6 oz.jar marinated artichoke hearts, drained and diced fine

¼ tsp hot pepper sauce

Melba toast or whole grain crackers (optional)

Directions:

Remove any shells or cartilage from crab.

Place all Ingredients in a small crock pot. Cover and cook on high 1 ½ - 2 hours, or until heated through and cream cheese is melted. Stir after 1 hour.

Serve with Melba toast or whole grain crackers. Serving size is ¼ cup.

Nutrition:

Calories 106 Total Carbs 7g Net Carbs 6g Protein 5g Fat 8g Sugar 3g Fiber 1g

46   Cranberry & Almond Granola Bars

Preparation time: 15 minutes

Cooking time: 20 minutes

Servings: 12

Ingredients:

1 egg

1 egg white

What you'll need from store cupboard:

2 cup low-fat granola

¼ cup dried cranberries, sweetened

¼ cup almonds, chopped

2 tbsp. Splenda

1 teaspoon almond extract

½ tsp cinnamon

Directions:

Heat oven to 350 degrees. Line the bottom and sides of an 8-inch baking dish with parchment paper.

In a large bowl, combine dry Ingredients including the cranberries.

In a small bowl, whisk together egg, egg white and extract. Pour over dry Ingredients and mix until combined.

Press mixture into the prepared pan. Bake 20 minutes or until light brown.

Cool in the pan for 5 minutes. Then carefully lift the bars from the pan onto a cutting board. Use a sharp knife to cut into 12 bars. Cool completely and store in an airtight container.

Nutrition:

Calories 85 Total Carbs 14g Net Carbs 13g Protein 3g Fat 3g Sugar 5g Fiber 1g

47   Crispy Baked Cheese Puffs

Preparation time: 5 minutes

Cooking time: 10 minutes

Servings: 4

Ingredients:

2 eggs

½ cup cheddar cheese, grated

¼ cup mozzarella, grated

What you'll need from store cupboard:

½ cup almond flour

¼ cup reduced fat Parmesan

½ tsp baking powder

Black pepper

Directions:

Heat oven to 400 degrees. Line a baking sheet with parchment paper.

In a large bowl, whisk eggs until lightly beaten. Add remaining Ingredients and mix well.

Divide into 8 pieces and roll into balls. Place on prepared baking sheet. Bake 10-12 minutes or until golden brown. Serve as is or with your favorite dipping sauce.

Nutrition:

Calories 129 Total Carbs 2g Net Carbs 1g Protein 8g Fat 10g Sugar 0g Fiber 1g

48   Crunchy Apple Fries

Preparation time: 15 minutes

Cooking time: 10 minutes

Servings: 8

Ingredients:

3 apples, peeled, cored, and sliced into ½-inch pieces

¼ cup reduced fat margarine, melted

2 tbsp. walnuts, chopped

What you'll need from the store cupboard

¼ cup quick oats

3 tbsp. light brown sugar

2 tbsp. whole wheat flour

1 tsp cinnamon

1/8 tsp salt

Directions:

Heat oven to 425 degrees. Put a wire rack on a large cookie sheet.

Add oats and walnuts to a food processor or blender and process until the mixture resembles flour.

Place the oat mixture in a shallow pan and add brown sugar, flour, cinnamon, and salt, mix well. Pour melted butter in a separate shallow pan.

Dip apple slices in margarine, then roll in oat mixture to coat completely. Place on wire rack.

Bake 10 – 12 minutes or until golden brown. Let cool before serving.

Nutrition:

Calories 146 Total Carbs 20g Net Carbs 17g Protein 1g Fat 7g Sugar 13g Fiber 3g

49   Strawberry Popsicles

Preparation time: 10 minutes

Cooking time: 30 minutes

Servings: 6

Ingredients:

5 drops of Liquid Stevia

¼ cup Oats, old-fashioned, grounded

4 oz. Cottage Cheese, low-fat

Juice from 4 Lemons

1 ½ lb. Strawberries

Directions:

Add all the ingredients in a high-speed blender and blend until it becomes smooth.

Once pureed, pour the mixture to the popsicle molds and place it in the freezer overnight or for a minimum of 6 hours. Serve and enjoy.

Tip: Meyers lemon would be the best choice to use for lemons.

Nutrition: Calories: 73cal Carbohydrates: 12g Proteins: 3.5g Fat: 0.5g Sodium: 67mg

50   Chocolate Fudge

Preparation time: 10 minutes

Cooking time: 30 minutes

Servings: 12 Fudges

Ingredients:

¼ cup Pecans, chopped

1 cup Heavy Whipping Cream

1 cup Chocolate Chips, low-carb

1/3 cup Erythritol

1 tsp. Vanilla Extract

2 tbsp. Butter

Directions:

Heat a medium-sized pan and to this, stir in whipping cream, vanilla extract, butter, and erythritol.

Continue stirring for 15 minutes or until you get a slightly browned condensed milk with a thick texture.

Allow to cool for 12 minutes and then add the chocolate chips.

Once the chocolate chips have melted, pour the mixture to a parchment paper-lined loaf pan and top it with pecans.

Keep in the refrigerator for at least an hour or more.

Serve and enjoy.

Tip: Instead of pecans, you can use any pecans.

Nutrition: Calories: 154.77cal Carbohydrates: 10.79g Proteins: 1.87g Fat: 15.5g Sodium: 29mg

Conclusion

Diabetes can be managed and treated effectively, although the process of doing so requires knowledge, discipline, patience and passion. Your health and happiness does not have to drop along with your insulin and blood glucose levels. In fact, you can make your life even better if you learn as much as you can about how your body functions as a diabetic and follow a healthy lifestyle suitable for diabetics.

Most of the successful management of diabetes relies on the right food choices, and getting enough exercise. Diabetes is a long term condition which you will have to deal with for the rest of your life, but you can lead a full and active life when you are armed with the knowledge you need to understand and manage your condition.

Hypoglycemia is an ever present concern for diabetics. That's when the blood sugar levels drop dangerously low, and weight loss diets and too much exercise can cause a hypoglycemic incident. In fact, just about everything about diabetes revolves around blood glucose levels, so it's important that you understand how to keep these levels stable.

Diabetes in itself is not necessarily life-threatening, but there can be complications as a result of the condition and again, most of these complications can be attributed to fluctuating blood glucose levels, which can cause a lot of stress to the system. Most of the complications associated with diabetes – including diabetic neuropathies, retinal neuropathy, heart disease, high blood pressure and high cholesterol – can be prevented or controlled by keeping blood glucose levels within the healthy range.

Knowledge is power, so make sure you learn as much as possible about the treatment and management of diabetes, particularly how it affects you as an individual, because every diabetes journey is unique. What works for your friend or neighbor may not necessarily be the right thing for you. Make friends with and make use of your health care providers, because they can help you to manage your condition effectively. They have seen all the complications and permutations, and they know how to address your concerns and help you through the bad spells and the down times. No matter how well you manage your diabetes, there will be times when nothing seems to go right, and you feel unwell, afraid and alone. The support of your family and your medical team will help you through those times.

Always wear your medical ID, and make sure that people you work with and socialize with know that you are diabetic, and what to do should you become ill. It's particularly important to notify the instructor if you attend an exercise class or the gym, so that they can take appropriate action to get you the treatment you need as quickly as possible should you have problems.

CPSIA information can be obtained
at www.ICGtesting.com
Printed in the USA
BVHW040300280421
605952BV00015B/2371

9 781801 656597